To seek out the facts,

Finally confront the truth,

And to pass it on.

J.A.M. (2015)

PUBLISHER'S NOTE

This book has been written through the uniquely bias lens of one individual, myself. The names of people, certain recollections and specific personal identifying details have been slightly altered and/or removed to ensure privacy and anonymity.

It must be kept in mind that one delivery driver can see almost five hundred patients in any given month spanning across dozens of cities, so the chances any of these stories being about you, or someone you know, are highly doubtful.

Or is it?

--------- *Thank you Robyn for taking the time to edit* ----------

The Kindest in California – Confessions of a Medical Marijuana Delivery Driver

Copyright © Jeff A. Meints, November 2015

ISBN#

INDEX

CHAPTER 1

Daily Deliveries into your Home . . . . *Page 6*

CHAPTER 2

Patients, A-Z . . . . *Page 29*

CHAPTER 3

Bigger Picture – Relief . . . . *Page 88*

CHAPTER 4

Confessions of a

Medical Marijuana Delivery Driver . . . . *Page 93*

CHAPTER 1

Daily Deliveries into your Home

The air conditioning of the car comforts me greatly as the outside heats attempts to penetrate my cryogenic chamber, unsuccessfully. I close my eyes and conserve energy for what's inevitably to come.

"BLING, BLING" my phone shouts at me, telling me that it is time to go. Thumbing over my phone, I look through the ticket confirming that the paperwork is all done so I input the zip code, address and then into drive I go.

Technology and simple gestures allow me to call ahead of time confirming my estimated time of arrival, usually within five to ten minutes, all the while steadily and safely maneuvering through life's traffic.

I've been told multiple times before I got this position and throughout my time at the position,

"The bar has been set low, so just do your job and you're golden."

This is why I start twenty minutes before my usual start time allowing me to spend a few extra minutes with each patient, if needed. Going that extra mile is worth it every time on many different levels.

I arrive within five minutes after receiving the ticket, most everyone loves punctuality, I retrieve my case from the trunk and walk up to the front door of this million dollar Del Mar home that overlooks the sparkling blue Pacific Ocean.

The doorbell notifies my patient through a series of "DONG DONG DONG DONG DOOOONGs" that I have arrived. It makes me feel briefly special. The doorbell silences and a flurry of yips, yaps, woofs and aroos fills the silence.

"Dogs, great," I think sarcastically.

Don't get me wrong, I grew up with dogs from childhood, bit in the face twice, I trained dogs during one of my first jobs out of high school at the Human Society and overall, I love dogs... but rarely in these instances do dogs, behave.

The door opens and we exchange introductions over the chorus of Mrs. Chihuaha and Mr.Pitbull. My patient inquires if I was ok with dogs followed by the historically infamous statement,

"They are very well behaved and very nice."

I rarely have issues, so I acknowledge that they can stay.

The pitbull was the stereotypical lapdog, despite its enormous size, with a beautiful joker-face smile and it definitely had not been trained the command, "Down." The Pit-Bull's partner in crime was this non-stop yipping and yapping little Chihuahua that also possessed another wonderful quality: Bitey-ness.

By the time I walked into the living room with my case I had already been nipped on the back of my ankles twice by the over-territorial little Napoleon. I always kept quiet about these things because these visits were usually short and somewhat brief, unless through indecision or if it was a new patient who had a lot of questions.

"Dispatch told me that you are a New Patient and you have some questions for me. I will go through my case with you, go over our coupons and then figure out what you want."

I open my sheath and slide out my display case setting it upon the living room table directly in front of her. Many earthly aromas fill the air and I begin.

"Every driver will be different. Some might have their case well stocked, depending on the day and time of day. Some drivers might have their case organized and some might not. Mine however, is organized. On the far right of my case is all the Sativa strains, the middle is my Hybrid strains and the far left is my Indica strains. All our bottles are pre-weighed out to three point eight grams, where as any normal eighter is usually three point five grams and it is also marked on the top right of the label. The bottom right of the bottle label is our donation fee and the top left of the bottle label is the strain."

I pause briefly and the patient nods with wide eyes, so I continue,

"My case has everything from pre-rolls, hash bullets, Cavi-Cones, Korova edibles, Cheeba Chews, crumbles, shatters and oils, CBD products, oral strips, transdermal patches and so much more. Now to the best part... our coupons. There is our daily DOGO, should have a T in there somewhere, which is buy three eighters and get the fourth eighter free. You can mix and match with prices, but the cheapest is always the freebie. The eighters can be anywhere from mid-shelf fourty dollar on up to top shelf sixty dollar eighters. So if you got all sixties then it would be only one hundred eighty for four top shelf eighters. Oh yeah, there is also a ten percent off for seniors, veterans and the disabled daily discount which you can stack with the DOGO."

My patient smiles and says,

"Wow, that's a great deal."

Making eye-contact with my patient I smile enthusiastically and say,

" There is also the Weedmaps coupon deal which changes every day, so always ask your driver, *"What is the Weedmaps Deal for the day?"* Otherwise your driver might forget. Today for example, the Weedmaps coupon is do a fourty dollar donation and receive a free Trainwreck, which is a Sativa strain and actually smells and smokes amazing. Here see for yourself."

I hand the patient a pre-weighed three point eight gram medicine bottle filled with the Sativa strain, Trainwreck. My patient opens the bottle and inhales the fragrance to test the quality. My patient looks over the strain while I finish plugging the final two coupons.

"You are also getting a five-hole punch card to be used over the course of five deliveries, whenever you want. It won't stack with the Weedmaps Deal, but it will stack with the DOGO deal. And finally, we have a Return Policy."

My patient puts the lid back on the bottle and places it back into the spot in the case.

"A Return Policy?! No Way!"

"Yup, you really can't lose with us. All our drivers are hourly paid so when I recommend something or not it is probably because that is my opinion on it. I've heard of horror stories from other patients about delivery services that are commission based. Way to cutthroat. I love this company. Best company I've ever worked for and I know you will be satisfied too."

I pause briefly before asking my patient,

"So enough of my blah, blah. What were you looking for today?"

Relief

This should be about the moment where you have come to the realization that I am a medical marijuana delivery driver. Well that and the fact it is the title of this book.

Yup, for ten hours a day, five too six days a week I drive anywhere from the Camp Pendleton area on down to Del Mar, Poway and up through Vista into Oceanside. I'm paid minimum wage, a whoppin' eleven dollars an hour, plus twenty dollars for gas a day.

In one year I have driven over thirty thousand miles, I have met and now know intimately hundreds of Californian medical marijuana patients and have spent thousands of dollars to keep my vehicle on the road delivering to these amazing people.

I'm Californian born, adopted and bred, and looking back on those thirty five years perhaps it was obvious that I would eventually end up working a position like this.

Armed to the teeth and protected only by my official California State stamped and sealed medical marijuana card issued by the San Diego Health and Human Services Agency, a tiny binder of legal documents in the event of police interaction, the contents of my trunk and a constant environmental awareness that keeps me on guard.

Rarely there will be days where I only see one or two patients in a ten hour period then there are those days where I have delivered to over twenty five patients in an eight hour work day all while avoiding everything life has to throw at me from potholes, people, putzs and police.

I'm not even the only driver, nor is there only one route. Some routes stretch as far north as the Fresno area while the majority of the deliveries are down here in beautiful Southern California. All of the above does not even account for all of our growing competition scattered across California and nationwide.

The demand for relief is high, no pun intended.

Relief of all kinds.

Reliefs such as the stress-relief of parenting,

schooling, work to family, finances, friend, love, life and death.

Despite the scientific fact that stress kills these reliefs are usually debated away as reliefs one should handle without assistance, however the financial success and overwhelming demand for the pharmaceutical industry and local brewers contradict that self assistance or self coping debate.

The more common reliefs I encounter that my patients suffer from are life debilitating and sometimes, life-ending ailments.

Some patients have just been diagnosed or have gone through or are going through rehabilitation or treatments, such as chemotherapy while some of my patients are in remission and others are being re-diagnosed and starting chemotherapy for a second or third time.

There is a dire need in the world today for any avenue of relief, even if temporary, such as losing your loved one, having just gotten married, or the physical, mental and emotional strain taken on from recently having a baby. All are situations that require some form of relief.

I've seen patients who have Lime disease, Fibromyalgia, Krohn's, Alzheimer's, cancer of all types, Narcolepsym Rubella Syndrome and more. I have seen a buffet of pain and suffering that all happens to be relieved through the medicine that is within my case. I receive "God Bless what you do" comments frequently and I sometimes get tipped pretty well all the while watching my patient's attitude and demeanor change for the better. This daily gratitude and relief that I encounter is what reminds me that I am doing a good thing.

"Every driver is different" is a managed expectation I always leave each patient with because on any given time of day my role as a driver can easily change and every driver has their own way of doing things.

I have been and continue to be a driver but I have also played the role of nutritionist, counselor, salesman, and I treat all my patients as if they were my family and as if they were my friend recommending to them what I think will benefit their specific situation and ailment.

Going that extra mile to provide proper relief, even if no tip or acknowledgement is received, is always worth it.

Dispatch

Dispatch is the brain of our daily dealings from getting emails, phone messages and calls to interacting with every type of personality that exists out there in the world. Patients who are disgruntle, happy, in pain, lonely and who are simply obnoxious are on a daily basis, making Dispatch's life quite interesting, to say the least.

I have heard stories of Dispatch being cussed out by patients and some patients have gone so far as to bring a Dispatcher to tears through verbal abuse. Of course once a delivery driver shows up all that bully-courage the patient had over the phone vanishes and all that remains is a fellow human being seeking relief. Dispatch definitely deserves acknowledgement for the amount of patients they handle a day and what they have to go with during some of those interactions.

The most powerful people in a driver's life is Dispatch. Dispatch can wittingly or unwittingly make a driver's day smooth and easy or beyond hellish. The best bet is to never get on a dispatcher's bad side, and for me that is easy, because I love Dispatch.

Dangers

My job is in no way easy, safe, fun, or simple.

Daily dangers can include everything from being robbed, kidnapped, unknowingly entering an unsafe home or situation, interactions with law enforcement, mentally or emotionally unstable patients, dogs that attack, but my number one daily danger is driving.

Just about every day within my ten hour work shift I avoid two to three minor accidents and if I am lucky only two to three major accidents a week. The tension created through these daily near misses can be physically and mentally exhausting.

Robbed

There have only been a few robberies I have heard of through the grapevine over the past four years.

One story was of a driver who was put into his trunk and thankfully, later found safe with all of his medicine stolen.

I accumulated bits and pieces of the most recent robbery where a female driver was leaving a patient's apartment one evening. It was very dark in the parking lot while she walked towards her car, case in one hand and phone in the other.

Two Hispanic men approached her quickly, one attempted to put her into a headlock and the other grabbed the case.

She quickly wriggled free and ran into the darkness, stealthily hiding in some bushes while they yelled after her,

"Leave your keys."

She obviously did not respond and hid until she thought it was safe to call for assistance. After assistance arrived, they found her car had been ransacked and all the medicine taken.

Semi-Trucks

My second month on the job, I was stuck in traffic in gorgeous Del Mar, so it wasn't that big of a deal. It was a two lane road with the Del Mar racetrack on the left hand side. It was a long line of cars waited for the red light and I was the very last person in this long line.

Then there was the intensely loud sound of semi-brakes locking and tires screeching echoing through the air.

A semi-truck soars past the left side of my car into the oncoming traffic lane in order to avoid slamming in the back of me, as smoke and the smell of burning rubber fills in the air.

Thankfully there was no traffic coming which allowed the semi-truck driver to make this maneuver safely, for everyone.

But still, that was way to close.

Motorcycles and Bicycles

I have found that some of the most entitled entities on the road are motorcycle drivers and bicyclists.

Only in California will you find motorcycle riders driving down the middle lanes and off into the bicycle lanes simply to get to where they are going a few minutes quicker, despite the risk to themselves and others.

They are the risk takers that I see daily on the road and I envy other states that have laws in place that prevent motorcycles from driving down the middle lanes, as they are allowed to do here legally in California.

Bicyclists are way too trusting, or are not fully grasping the fact that you cannot trust other drivers on the road to notice your spandex stealthy self, especially on a two lane, no-bike lane highway with a cliff on one side and a mountain on the other with a speed limit of 55 miles per hour.

Bicyclists rarely stop at stop signs, rarely use hand motions to indicate to drivers they are about to venture into the middle of the road and turn and I have witnessed numerous Del Mar bicyclists road rage on cars from spitting, throwing objects and slamming vehicles with the fists all in the heat of the moment.

Rain, Sleet, Wind and Heat

While most California days are filled with sunshine, waves, beautiful people and lollipops most that live in California really know how truly schizophrenic our weather really is.

From extreme heat, frigid cold, pouring down rain that leads to slick roads, floods, sink holes and car accidents, hurricane like winds that try to push cars into each other and hail that can almost crack a windshield.

Pedestrians

Pedestrians are quite interesting these days as they take no heed to where a crosswalk is located and instead cross at any time they chose. I have witnessed pedestrians practically jump into oncoming traffic. Each time I think to myself,

"These people have not played the old-school video game "Frogger" and they need to."

People's lack of spatial awareness is ever present these days.

Hourly Pay + Tips – Risk versus Reward

It is difficult to weigh the risk versus reward with this position.   I only get paid eleven dollars an hour plus twenty dollars for gas, per day. This is not accounting the wear and tear on my car equating to thousands of dollars within the first year for repairs from the ten hours of driving a day. Also not considered is every day without an accident or incident.

The other end of the scale is the relief I bring my patients.

The relief I bring to my patients on a daily basis is priceless. I learn about these patients lives, I meet their family members, friends and pets, their talents, and I provide a service that is truly unique and worthwhile.

There also is something liberating to being in a position of almost complete autonomy, but there is also the issue of law enforcement. Despite having all my paperwork and license the police can easily make my life beyond inconvenient.

I have only been pulled over once in my year of delivering and my citation was, ironically, tailgating.

More specifically, the officer claimed that I was tailgating him.

CHAPTER 2

Patients, A-Z

While I am sure I missed many different types of Patients in this A-Z listing I just hope what I have come up with through my travels and what I have written down here enlightens, brings a little insight, maybe a smile, and legitimacy into the world of medical marijuana.

AGREEABLE PATIENTS

These patients are by far the easiest patients I have come across. They are the type of patient that will get whatever you recommend even when they do not want it.

Despite them being agreeable to whatever you recommend, be wary with your recommendations because these patients will remember your failed recommendation and will request to Dispatch that you no longer deliver to that particular patient.

AILMENTS OF PATIENTS

By far the most common type of patient that I have encountered is patients with life changing, altering and/or debilitating ailments.
Cancer is the most common of these ailments yet branches out to so many differing cancers that it is mind boggling. The most common cancer I have come across that my patients suffer from is lymphoma, testicular, brain and skin cancer.

I have lime disease patients, narcoleptic, schizophrenic and an endless array of many other varying physical, mental and emotional ailments. Arthritis, body pains, headaches, migraines…. The patients I visit regularly always find great relief in my visits.

Those recovering from strokes, heart attacks, needing to lower their blood pressure, reduce or stop epileptic episodes, these patients are turning towards medical marijuana for relief from their ailment.

Addiction from pharmaceutical drugs is another common ailment I come across. Patients that have been on certain pharmaceuticals for so long that they are now using medical marijuana to allow their body to repair from all the side effects brought on from the pharmaceuticals.

There are many recovering addicts from drugs such as heroin, cocaine and even alcohol that are turning to medical marijuana for their relief instead of the detrimental dead end that those other substances can lead to.

The majority of my patients inform me of their medical history even though most of the time I do not inquire. This can be incredibly helpful to the educated medical marijuana delivery driver allowing the driver to cater that delivery experience specifically to that patient so they can pick out the proper flower strains or edibles or oils or balms that will bring relief to their specific ailment.

ANGRY PATIENTS

While the angry patient might have many negative things to say, scowls and frowns galore and more complaints than compliments it is easy to lose sight of the fact that these are patients and are seeking relief from some type of ailment, which might be the reason they are so angry.

It is important to try and keep an open mind with each patient and an understanding that you do not know what they are going through in life, which could be causing the way they are acting. They just might be in intense pain and have very little avenues of relief, and that is where I come in.

Then there are those patients who are just naturally angry and there is very little I can do in those situations other than be my charming self.

ATHLETES

A few of my patients are avid supporters of consuming medical marijuana before going on their long bike rides, or jogging, or hitting the gym and I have even met an amazingly intelligent and talented surfer chick who almost has her Master Degree in medicine and is planning on becoming a doctor.

BEAUTICIANS

From hairstylists, manicurists, to make-up artists there is no denying the long hours and tedious hard work that goes into making us look beautiful on a daily basis require relief just like any other worker.

BOTANISTS

I have a few patients that are Professors at local colleges and they teach Botany. These patient's houses usually have greenhouses and their yards are absolutely gorgeous with rare and exotic plants blooming daily.

Some patients have walked me through their greenhouses showing me various, some familiar, plants and other patients have provided me tips on hydroponics.

<u>CAREGIVERS</u>

When patients are unable to travel to physical dispensaries or are unable to interact or be involved with medical marijuana deliveries is usually when a Caregiver comes in. Sometimes patients are completely incapacitated and even require assistance from their Caregivers to take their medications.

A spouse, family member or friend can obtain a Caregiver's License allowing them to obtain medical marijuana for whoever is designated upon their license. Whoever they are assisting with their medical needs must also have a medical marijuana recommendation along with their

Caregiver's name upon that license, in most cases.

One such patient that I have is a Caregiver for her sister who has Rubella Syndrome. She has been blind, deaf and mute since she was born, and she is seventy five years old now. For her whole life she has never see a face, never heard a sound and has never been able to speak to anyone, and I have come to realize that there is nothing sad about it.

This for her is normal everyday life and it is beyond fascinating to meet her. She can sense vibrations and can maneuver within her own home but as far as how she interprets and perceives those vibrations and her surroundings will forever be a mystery.

CBD-ONLY PATIENTS

More and more patients are transitioning to CBD only products that have little-to-no THC, therefore will provide no medicating effects to the patient.

This daily CBD regiment should be thought of as any other nutritional supplement, and should be taken every day otherwise it will provide no beneficial effects in the long run.

Out of all the CBD products I have come across the most beneficial in both price and quantity is the CBD Tincture.

One tincture lasts a patient one month at a low $45.00 a bottle where-as any other CBD only product is usually only one dose for some high cost.

Remember, CBD is not a cure-all, so do not break the bank buying these products.

CHILDREN OF PATIENTS

While children cannot yet obtain a medical marijuana recommendation in California there are still plenty of kid interactions during deliveries and when going into the home of a patient it is only natural to occasionally encounter children.

There is nothing cuter and amusing than a parents varying reaction when a toddler waddles into the room where my patient and I are picking out what medicine they want from my case. The parent, usually, immediately scoops up the baby to return it to the parent in the other room inquiring as to how a prison escape occurred while apologizing repeatedly with a cherry-red face.

Personally I do not mind if a patient's children are in the room because nothing is going on that they shouldn't know about but it is the patient's house. In the end, whatever makes my patient's most comfortable is the route I always take.

Then there are the parents who do not mind their children being in the room and they treat it like it should be treated, which is a medical delivery and an educational moment.

"Daddy's getting his medicine," is a very honest reason commonly given to the kiddos.

Quite a few of these kids know me on a first name basis and I have had a few actually tell me how much it helps their mom or dad.

"Daddy's much nicer when he has his medicine."

COOKING PATIENTS

So many wonderful offers through the months of the most gloriously looking and smelling food ever dreamed. These patients have a tendency to provide me on my visits with an endless array of cultural delights and culinary conjured treats that my nose, mouth and senses always enjoy, and always remember.

CREATIVE/ARTISTIC PATIENTS

I have seen sunrises, sunsets and glowing moons illuminating foreign shores upon canvas, cities and fortresses of LEGOs, a robotics lab out of the back of a garage and gorgeously manicured and landscaped properties, all done by the creative hands and minds of my patients.

COMPASSIONATE PATIENTS

One amazing thing about the company that I work for is that they offer their patients the option to be a "Compassionate Patient" which requires them to fill out a form and present documentation describing their ailment or ailments and the need for financial assistance.   If approved then the patient has a weekly allowance providing them free deliveries and free medicine for each week.

Those deliveries are by far the most enlightening because each time you visit that specific Compassionate Patient you learn more and more about them, their lives, their families and their ailment. It is a unique feeling knowing how much relief you are bringing to someone who suffers so greatly and so very little effort was required to make this happen.

DIVORCED PATIENTS

I have gotten to know many patients to the point where one day I am delivering to a new address and I know the name looks familiar, but the address is different. Maybe Dispatch screwed something up on their end.

Once I arrive and I see their face and realize that they have either traded up, and I am now delivering to a house or mansion versus the apartment I had delivered to for months.

A couple times those once married patients who both lived in a house or mansion are suddenly all by themselves and I am delivering to their new address at an apartment.

I can relate to being with someone for almost ten years and then giving everything to your now parting partner leaving yourself with just a car and a shattered dream.

DOCTORS

Not only do doctors recommend to their patients to use medical marijuana, but some of these doctors are also my patients.

EDIBLE PATIENTS

There are many patients transitioning to edibles instead of smoking flower or concentrates. Some patients want to give their lungs a break while other patients require more medicating and edibles can pack a serious punch.

What I have learned after eating a one thousand milligram Korova brownie one of my days off.

When consuming an edible it usually will activate at about the hour mark so remember these tips:

A) Do not consume the complete edible if it is high in milligrams. Think of it as a pill and you will need to figure out your dosage and regiment it appropriately. Start at a low milligram, such as ten milligrams of THC.

B) Always have or get food into your stomach soon after eating the edible. This will keep your digesting going and it should prevent any stomach issues.

C) Take a cool shower in the event of any heart racing or sweats. It might resemble an anxiety attack. The cool water will reset your body temperature.

D) Never go to sleep immediately after eating an edible. It will not digest and when you wake up it will kick in all at once and it might feel like an anxiety attack. If this occurs, crawl to the shower and you should be good.

ELDERLY PATIENTS

The elderly are always interesting patients. The diversity of these patients can range anywhere from the elderly couple who have been together since high school, the very wealthy single elderly person who somehow is more active than kids in high school, the very shy and inexperienced elderly who have never used medical marijuana before, the elderly with a laundry list of ailments that they are attempting to relieve.

These elderly patients are always polite, they tip well and there are rarely ever any awkward moments. In fact, some drivers get care packages from these elderly patients such as granola bars, water, candy and more. It is almost as if we have been adopted by an army of grandparents.

ENHANCEMENT PATIENTS

The 1998 movie titled Half Baked covered this type of patient beautifully through the actor John Stewart.

> *"You ever seen the back of a twenty dollar bill man? Have you ever seen the back of a twenty dollar bill.... On weed?!"*

> *~John Stewart, 1998, Half Baked*

Essentially, an enhancement patient is someone who believes that any activity, while on medical marijuana, makes that particular activity far greater.

EX-CONS

These are some of the more colorful patients I come across and I mean colorful through their very colorful and unique tattoos. Most of these patients have a "give respect in order to receive respect" attitude which makes them easy to work with.

FLIGHT ATTENDANTS

These patients have stories from near and far that can are usually hilarious and diverse, and most often these patients are in a little high strung and are on the way out the door to travel somewhere new.

FORGETFUL PATIENTS

Patients have been asleep when I have arrived, surprised that they had a delivery, or they have forgotten their money requiring me to return later to finish the delivery and there even have been some who have cancelled the delivery right there on the spot due to their forgetfulness.

FOUR TWENTY PATIENTS

Some patients have a daily ritual that dictates they must medicate at the time 4:20 on the clock. It does not matter if it is in the p.m. or a.m., or if the time really is 4:20, because that specific time is the universal timeframe for Cannabis smokers worldwide.

Surprisingly I do not receive many delivers at this time each day and in a way it is kind of disappointing.

GAMERS

There are patients who rarely play, who weekly play to those who live and breathe games of all types from Dungeon and Dragons, X-Box, Playstation, Wii, LARPERs to P.C. gamers and more. There is no gamer I can think of that I have not come across.

GREEN PATIENTS

I have been privileged enough to tour a half acre plot of land while on a delivery to a patient that had a tiny fifty foot wind turbine that cost only ten thousand dollars ten years ago. It provided my patient's whole house unlimited power, always gave energy back to the grid and he gets money back each month from the power company.

Solar power is becoming more popular and I see it being installed on my patient's homes more and more. I see these trends all over San Diego county in varying socioeconomic groups.

GROUPS

Groups of Men

For some reason groups of guys usually display a pack mentality. Some of these groups of men act like packs of wolves or apes but overall there is always an alpha of the group. The boisterous individual who is always standing, talking loudly, usually in your face, and asks questions, such as,

"Aren't you afraid of getting jacked and all your stuff taken?"

Laughter follows from the pack, perhaps to relieve any tension or maybe to create it. I have responded to this territorial question in the past with,

"Naw, no fear at all. I know where you live."

Each time this response has been followed by further laughter and I, each time, temporarily claim the Alpha role of that pack.

There has only been two times that things have been stolen out of my case without my knowledge. Each time was when interacting with a group of guys.

They have a sneaky routine that goes like this:

> Usually while one person distracts you by looking at the products in your case or by asking you a question while the other person with a quick-hand, Houdini's a bottle, or some other product.

Unfortunately, you never realize these moments of theft until inventory is taken days later or if you manage to notice that extra empty slot after taking your case back to your car, but by the end you will be paying out of your own pocket for your mistake.

Groups of Women

Groups of females tend to be more welcoming and very receptive to new information. Women tend to be, at times, giggly, inquisitive and even flirty. Obviously here is safety in numbers providing the patient a more comfortable setting compared to when they are by themselves with a stranger who they just met and invited into their home to acquire medicinal marijuana.

It is always flattering when the patient requests if you can be their personal driver at the end of a smooth delivery but again, a driver must wonder if this interest is genuine in a professional or non-professional way. In those flirty moments a driver could easily become involved with a patient on an intimate level and if so, that patient could simply be using the driver to get close to the product. It is difficult to know someone's intentions these days when so many people are seeking relief from some ailment.

HIPPIES

From long-haired hippies to dred-lock Rastafarians, one thing with these patients that always remains the same, aside from the scent of incense in the air, is a beyond welcoming and positive attitude with every delivery.

HONEST PATIENTS

One evening I lost my money bag near the end of an exhausting ten hour shift. It was 11 p.m. and I drove wearily back to my last two patients. Upon arriving at the first dark and lonely street I hear a hissing in the darkness after exiting my car to check the ground for the cash bag.

My front car tire was going flat.

After finding nothing at the two patients house I barely managed to crawl into a gas station riding on the rim of my tire.

I paid four hundred dollars out of my own pocket to cover my mistake.

Three days later a patient calls and says he received a call from a man who found a bag with a check and money in it. My four hundred dollars was returned to my bank account and I was beyond grateful that our company accepts checks.

That honest patient received a free eighter and my eternal gratitude.

HUNG-OVER

Try not to talk too loud during these deliveries, because as the patient has reminded you a few times now, they went out drinking last night. Usually these patients have kids going crazy in the house, yelling and screaming, and you can just tell this patient wants nothing more than to take a nap.

INSOMNIAC PATIENTS

Can you imagine only sleeping four hours a day? Some of my patients have come to the painful realization that pharmaceuticals and alcohol possess detrimental side effects when using in order to sleep. Hangovers and other inner issues arise making those two above options not a solution, but an increase in the already existing problem.

When I wake up every morning at 2 a.m. the first thing I do is reach for my Indica strain and back to sleep I go within minutes versus within hours. No hangover, no residual effects after waking up, just rested and ready for the day.

INTOXICATED

"I love you bro" is a common phrase when frequenting bars with your friends. It is always a little awkward when you just met a new patient who is beyond tipsy, already medicated, or "high" on any known or unknown substance. Most commonly the patient requests you just, "Pick out what you think is best," otherwise they can easily make the delivery unbearable through indecisiveness and by dragging it out. Confusion over money is quite typical during these deliveries combined with a sense of distrust often the question arises,

"How much money did I just give you?"

JERKFACES to JERRY SPRINGERS

Some rare patients, no matter how many coupons you stack up and how much money you save them, will forever act like jerkfaces.

These jerkfaces can be anywhere from rude, racist, sexist with inappropriate comments towards you or towards the world beyond the walls of their home.

Then there is the Jerry Springers who provide scenes out of the show. Tossing furniture, broken objects and screaming couples all the while you are trying to get the patient to pick out his medications.

Sometimes it gets so crazy you find yourself wondering if you need to pick a side and throw a chair.

LOTTO WINNER PATIENT

Yes, I have had one lottery winner patient. He had the huge check on his chair and he was celebrating it up with his first delivery with me. He almost cleaned my case out and he talked about how he never thought he would own a house and now it is possible. I have not seen him in months and I hope he is doing well.

KINDEST PATIENTS

There are countless patients who are beyond kind and who I enjoy seeing any day of the week.

KLEPTO PATIENTS

I had a paragraph here but the ever-so-rare klepto patient snagged it when I was on my coffee break.

MARRIED PATIENTS

There are many married patients I see weekly. Some married couples both have their recommendation while others only one partner does.

In these instances the partner without a recommendation usually has a job that they fear will persecute them for their medical needs, so they avoid getting a recommendation to avoid that persecution.

MARTIAL ARTIST PATIENTS

Patients that are trained in the sword, knife, bow, and hand-to-hand to those just beginning, I have seen an array of martial artists.

MILITARY PATIENTS

I have many military patients all from which suffer from a variety of ailments, but the most common that I encounter is Post Traumatic Stress Disorder.

NAKED PATIENTS

While I have not personally had the honor, or horror of a delivery of this nature I have heard a few stories of drivers who have arrived to patients with no clothes on. Thankfully these are rare instances.

NEWBEES

My all-time favorite patients are New Patients or as I think of them, "Newbees." These patients have never experienced our company before and in some cases, have never experienced a medical marijuana delivery service before.

This entails inviting a stranger into your home with the intention of donating towards their collective to acquire medical marijuana. To some this might be a little nerve wracking, awkward and maybe even beyond uncomfortable, but this is one example of the steps people are taking to find relief and the need to legalize it nationally.

First encounters or first time introductions are a very important thing. This sets the tone for all deliveries to follow or not. This blank slate allows me to inform and educate accurately and with ease. Most introductions usually take me about one to two minutes and that includes me covering my entire case, varying products and prices, our amazing flower return policy and most importantly, our company's daily coupons.

Some newbees can be quite quick-tempered and to-the-point, "I know what I want and I don't want to hear about anything else." It is up to the driver to take the time, or to not take the time, to then somehow eloquently insert,

"Ok, you definitely can have that and if you don't want to hear about the other coupons, which by the way can sometimes be a free eighter, then I guess I shall be on my way."

This usually gets the patient's attention and they become quite receptive. After-all, who doesn't want to save a few dollars or get a freebie on almost every delivery because it is hard enough to afford food these days, especially combined with our daily medical needs.

NO MONEY AND/OR ARE NOT HOME

To this day, I cannot wrap my brain around this repetitious scenario:

A patient calls to arrange a delivery or to make an a specific appointment time for a delivery and is told an estimated time of arrival, usually within the hour.

That patient is called within ten minutes of being informed and informs the patient that they should arrive within ten minutes.

The delivery driver arrives to find either the patient not home and they are out getting money, or the patient is home but they do not have the money for the delivery, which means they now have to leave to go get the money.

Now don't get me wrong, if a patient sets an appointment for a specific set delivery time, obviously that is when the delivery driver should arrive. That is an appointment.

But to not be home after you have already talked to me and were informed that I would be at your home within ten minutes…. Well that just drives me bonkers.

O.G.'s

"I've smoked ever since I was six years old! I know everything there is to know about weed!"

This is the most comical statement that I come across in my travels and I have titled this crowd the "Old School" patients.

These patients range in ages from 45 on up to 97 years old. Yes, I have a 97 year old patient. Each of these patients has a specific strain in mind that they remember smoking once long ago and they remember how much it impressed them like it was yesterday.

What is somehow lost upon these O.G.'s is that every batch of every strain is different than the last. That Blue Dream you smoked over twenty years ago is dramatically different than the Blue Dream that is in my case on any given day.

These O.G. patients are usually unreceptive to new products such as oils, vape pens, oral strips, waxes, transdermal patches and edibles. Most are strictly flower patients. However, with the right approach new information can easily be delivered and new avenues of relief attempted.

When you come across that O.G. patient who says, "I've only ever smoked flower," then toss in a question, such as, "Have you ever seen these new vape pens with THC oil? They are financially viable, discreet, smell almost sweet and are easy on your lungs."

If you pitch these new products right then patients everywhere will begin experiencing new and wonderful products that will bring them even more relief then they have experienced in the past.

ONLY THE LONELY

I would fall under this category if not for the fact that I rarely receive deliveries anymore due to my job.

There is an endless stream of patients who work day and night to the bone to just barely pay rent and barely fill their fridges. After those tiresome workdays one of the first things they do after they get off work is schedule a delivery and most times before they are even home.

Usually these patients are by themselves, living in a spacious, or cramped apartment or house, rarely with new stories about life and always will they ask before I depart,

"Wanna smoke a bowl before you go?"

Alas, professionalism and legalities prevent me from accepting these offers despite how appealing the invitation sounds. In these moments you can really tell that these patients just want someone to talk to and hang out with. I can relate.

OPTIMISTIC PATIENTS

Even on your worst day, these are the patients who always have something positive to say and it sometimes appears as if it never rains in their world, unless they want it to.

PESSIMISTIC PATIENTS

On the other side of that coin is our pessimistic patients who always have something to complain about whether it is politics, religion, the neighbors dog keeps pooping on their lawn, the flower is to dry or not potent enough, or that the weather is always too cold or too hot.

PETS AND ANIMALS, DOGS AND CATS, BIRDS, OH MY!

I consider myself an animal person not just because I grew up with numerous dogs, cats, fish, hamsters, turtles, lizards, snakes, rats and birds, nor because my first job was at the Escondido Humane Society where I overtime learned how to train dogs and other animals, but it is simply because I love animals and believe they are just about no different than human beings therefore should be treated with love, understanding and respect.

Ironically, my time at this position has led me to recall only the deliveries of pets misbehaving and acting like unruly children during my visits versus all the super cute and well behaved pets.

From being bitten several times in the back of the ankle while my patient insists,

"My dog is well behaved and is very nice,"

too the dog that has mud all over its paws and will not stop jumping all over you while the patient insists,

"He is never like this, he is usually so well behaved."

The most infamous of all time pet moments is the pet humping your leg moment and just recently I had a little Chihuahua named Taco attack my medicine case as I was leaving. Taco really wanted some meds apparently.

My most challenging pet moment was having two unruly, barking and jumping dogs combined with a screeching parrot. Every time I attempted to talk to my patient an explosion of barks and screeches obliterated my patient and I making it beyond impossible to communicate with each other. My ears were still ringing miles after leaving that house.

POLITICIANS AND PUBLIC OFFICIALS

This section has been deemed "don't ask, don't tell."

P.H.D. PROFESSORS

I have met many a P.H.D. Professor and I have even delivered to a Professor who used to teach me during my time at a community college.

PRISON GUARDS

Can you imagine having the job of prison guard? Beyond the risk to your life on a daily basis it is no doubt that the stress behind this job might require relief that pharmaceuticals and alcohol can never beneficially provide, which is where I come in.

QUESTIONS GALORE

The majority of patients have no questions unless it is about some new cool product that caught their eye in your case.

Usually when the questions galore patient pops up is during a "slammed" period when dozens of patients are in wait and even though you do not want to seem in a hurry, inside your head, it is time to hit the road.

RELIGIOUS

Sundays are usually quiet days up until church gets out. Almost usually around noon is when those quiet Sundays can become quite busy.

RECREATIONAL PATIENTS

While the general public stereotypically believes that the majority of medical marijuana patients are simply medicating recreationally versus for medical reasons.

I rarely come across recreational patients in my deliveries.

The majority of my patients are seeking out medication to alleviate some ailment or ailments they are burdened with. During my travels I have seen only a small percentage of recreational medical marijuana patients, but it is ironic that no matter the reason for using medical marijuana the end-result for all patients is always medical, whether they intended it that way or not.

By consuming medical marijuana in any form you are introducing into your body cannabidiol along with hundreds of other cannabis chemicals, called cannabinoids, that are highly beneficial to all human beings, so while you may think you are a recreational medical marijuana patient in reality you are receiving the same medical benefits as any other patient.

REVERSE PSYCHOLOGY PATIENTS

"What do you recommend?" is a very common question for patients to ask their delivery driver. Most patients listen to their drivers recommendations but there is always the other side of that coin.

Reverse psychology patients will ask you for your recommendation and always pick the opposite of what you recommend.

Sometimes I get the feeling that the patient thinks the delivery driver is receiving commission, hence his recommendations are not genuine.

If I get that feeling from the patient, that skepticism, I will usually inform the patient eloquently that all our drivers are hourly paid, which means we recommend what we like.

SMELL THOSE SMELLS

I haven't smoked cigarettes in years and thankfully there is no longer any desire. This lack of desire to smoke cigarettes is reinforced every time I deliver to cigarette smoking patients. No matter the amount of time spent with the patient, one minute or more, I always leave reeking of cigarettes. If you are a hand-shaking type of person then your hand will smell as if you just smoked a cigarette. Having a cigarette smoker as your first patient is not how I prefer to start my day.

Then there are those patients that just smell. Perhaps they do not believe in doing laundry, or showering, or cleaning up after their pets, or perhaps do not know how to clean and maybe in some cases, their noses simply just do not work any longer, but those patients are always a challenge because your nose and lungs have a tendency to deny you the breathes required to talk and stand upright.

Then there are the sweetest and most wonderful smelling scents and smells that ever drifted through the air.

Whether it is the patient's home that smells so beyond heavenly or it is the patient themselves there is no end to the perfumes, incenses and even an individual's natural scent, and that is why every patient, is a smelly patient in some way.

STRIPPER PATIENTS

Gorgeous, sexy, tone and tanned have been the theme of many of my stripper patients. I have had patients all glittered up and ready for "Pornstar night at the gentlemen's club" too just getting home from a long day.

Ironically, stripper patients do not know how to tip.

TATTOOED PATIENTS

Some of the most beautiful artwork I have seen in my travels is usually been upon the human body.

The most interesting part about my patient's tattoos is the stories behind them. Many have deeper meanings behind them and some have no meaning at all, but every patient's tattoos are always unique works of art.

TEACHERS

Many preschool, kindergarten, elementary, middle school and high school teachers are educated enough to know the many medical benefits to medical marijuana and that is probably why I have so many teachers as patients, aside from the stress of being an underpaid and overworked teacher.

TRANSGENDER

There any many transgender patients that I deliver to and I have gotten to know many of them very well.

It was interesting when you would call on the phone a patient with a female name, but a masculine voice would answer, so I naturally asked if the name of the female was there.

Thankfully each time these patients were polite and patient with my unknowingness.

Many of these patients discussed with me why they do not go out much and why they do not visit physical dispensaries. Once the people at the dispensary look at their I.D. and realize that the patient is transgender there is the possibility of being discriminated against and access to that particular dispensary denied.

I have heard some terrible stories of how these patients were treated.

UNDERCOVER COPS

There have been times during some deliveries where patients try to bend and break the rules, and these instances it could very well be possible that an undercover cop is trying to bust you.

Asking if a friend can participate in the delivery and it becomes obvious that the delivery is really for the friend and not your patient, or if they can do the delivery out of the back of my trunk, or if they can do the delivery out of the back of their work van are only a few ways a delivery driver can get himself into legal trouble.

A medical marijuana delivery driver must never make exceptions to the rules and laws in place. It is for the safety of the patient and the delivery driver.

If a patient will not agree to a legal setting or will not ask his guests to not participate in the delivery then no delivery will occur.

UNIFORMED PATIENTS

Very often, I have patients that are still wearing the uniforms of whatever job they have, when I arrive to perform the delivery.

I have seen uniforms, or work attire from Dominoe's Pizza Delivery, JC Penney, San Diego Credit Union, martial artist outfits, white coat lab tech assistant and even a clown costume.

UNKNOWING FAMILY, FRIENDS, LANDLORDS, NEIGHBORS, SPOUSE

The most entertaining patients, at least for me, are the patients who are focused on keeping their deliveries private or a secret.

Whether it is making sure the landlord doesn't see me arrive or depart, or it's the mother or father who won't be home for an hour, or the parents who are doing everything in their power to make sure their kids do not know. I have found that in the end secrecy means very little.

Sometimes this secrecy can turn this lawful and legal medical delivery into the appearance of a shady venture.

I have had deliveries where patients provide step-by-step instructions on where to park, when to call, what to do and not to do, where to wait until the patient signals. Keeping their deliveries private is incredibly important to these patients and that is why such extensive steps must sometimes be taken.

It is not uncommon for a lack of understanding in society to arise and discrimination to occur when it comes to medical marijuana.

However, once you have a family member or loved one who is suffering greatly and they find relief with medical marijuana the only question that remains for you to answer is,

"Will your pride over your opinion deny your loved one relief?"

VARYING RACES, SEXES, AGES, RELIGIONS AND CREEDS OF PATIENTS

Medical Marijuana discriminates against none and brings relief to patients of all races, sexes, ages, religions and creeds.

VEGAN PATIENTS

There are more and more edible vegan products popping up on the market and currently we carry a very tasty pack of pretzels that are incredibly moderate in dosage and ideal for the elderly who usually have lower tolerances.

VETERANARIAN PATIENTS

Many veterinarian patients have begun giving CBD-only products to their pets because they know the benefits CBD possesses.

What is ironic is that most of these patients do not take CBD on a daily basis themselves and treat their pets better than they are treating themselves.

VETERAN PATIENTS

There are countless patients who are veterans from wars dating all the way back to World War II. I have seen medals of all types, old black and white photos of past loved ones and historical events and war mementoes, such as sabers, knives and guns.

WAX PATIENTS

Wax patients, or "wax heads," as some have titled them, are only interested in wax products. This could be anything from wax crumbles, shatters, sap or honey consistency wax and sometimes other concentrates.

Wax is created through a varying chemical process that strips all the THC from the marijuana flower and turns it into one of the above types of wax. It is highly concentrated, far more potent than flower and only requires small dosages to medicate the patient.

WEALTHY PATIENTS

Million dollars homes, fancy cars and these patients always get their medicine in bulk, but they rarely tip and sometimes you do not even get a handshake.

WRITERS

Most of my writer patients have informed me that medical marijuana allows them to write with more ease. I agree with this sentiment and have always believed that a fluidity arises allowing creativity and our fingers to flow more easily.

YOGA INSTRUCTORS

There are a couple yoga instructor patients that are always beaming with positivity and energy. Most of them are usually already decked out in their Yoga gear and I have had the privilege of interrupting a session one evening.

X-RAY TECHNICIANS

If not for the fact that I actually have a patient that is an x-ray technician than I would not of had something for this section.

ZOOLOGISTS

These are patients with a passion for animals that is demonstrated through their careers and degrees. From working at local zoos to breeding endangered species and volunteering at the local Human Society, these patients are always full of life and joy.

CHAPTER 3

Bigger Picture – Relief

After working for over a year, ten hours a day, driving tens of thousands of miles to deliver to thousands of patients with varying ailments, all of which are seeking relief, a bigger picture starts to be painted.

The portrait appearing before our eyes is beyond the mere perception that cannabis is strictly recreational and has no medical value.

Varying ages from elderly to newborn adults find medical value through relief with no detrimental side effects. Medical marijuana is bringing relief and peace of mind to these patients when they could not achieve this degree of relief through other legitimate and accepted medical means.

Despite this ever present fact I encounter daily, there is plenty of discrimination towards these patients. There is discrimination towards those growing and harvesting cannabis, towards those establishments providing medical marijuana through licensed and legal means and discrimination towards the patients within all our communities that are simply seeking relief for some type of ailment.

The severity of our ailments should never come into question, nor should the degree of relief provided to our citizens. There should be no limit upon the relief distributed.

The lack of proper education regarding medical marijuana, industrial hemp and cannabis as a whole, stretches back into the

1900's starting with the Reefer Madness propaganda campaign combined with the Gore Files that were fake stories about cannabis use turned into newspaper articles that provided the misinformation and negative stereotypes that continue to mislead the public to this day.

What many people do not know is that in the 1930's, the American Medical Association supported medical marijuana and vocalized this support to Congress just before Congress criminalized Cannabis.

No "High" Cannabis Products

Alternatives now exist that contain little-to-no THC, therefore causes no "high" or psychoactive affect, through CBD-only products.

CBD, or cannabidiol is a naturally occurring chemical in all human beings.

All human beings, animals and some insects have an endocannibinoid system that is our bodies self defense system against disease, illness and injury. CBD regulates the homeostasis of our endocannabinoid system, so if our homeostasis is high then we can fight off disease, illness and heal from injuries more quickly, but if our homeostasis is low then we are more vulnerable to disease, illness and injury.

The last time we consumed CBD was in breast milk as a child, if we were even breast fed, so essentially we are depleted of CBD and our homeostasis low.

Cannabis is one of the only plants that produce CBD and now that the cannabis industry is evolving there are now CBD-only products on the market with high concentrations of CBD and little-to-no THC, so we can replenish our endocannibinoid system's homeostasis by using CBD as an essential everyday nutritional supplement.

Never should it be considered a cure-all.

I encourage everyone to research further into CBD, or cannibidiol, because only through public support, continued use of Cannabis products and further research can additional avenues of relief at an affordable cost be found for patients of all walks of life.

CHAPTER 4

Confessions of a Medical Marijuana Delivery Driver

"ARE YOU ONE OF THEM?!!"

When I received this particular patient's ticket I immediately recalled our first interaction.

It was around 10 p.m. and the first time I had visited this patient. I was instructed to not use the front door but the side door, to the left of the front door.

After knocking on the door to the left of the front door and no one came I proceeded to knock on each door to the left, waiting a brief period of time before moving on to the next door and knocking again. This process led me to discover that there were a couple different families living in this one house, and they did not seem to know who the heck my patient was. Was I even at the right house?

I soon found myself back at the front door, so I called the patient who was frustrated at me by this point and reinstructed me to the second door to the left of the front door. I knocked, waiting almost thirty seconds and finally my patient's girlfriend opened the door with a look of disdain on her face.

While that first delivery ended well our first interactions were awkward to say the least.

Thankfully I now knew what door to go to so I did not mess up and his girlfriend greeted me this time with a smile on her face. Everything went smooth all the way up until it was time to figure out my patient's total donation.

After punching everything into my phone that the patient was acquiring for the day, for some reason I decided in inquire if he knew anything about CBD products, since he was in a wheelchair and I felt CBD might help him.

My patient did not know anything about CBD or cannabadiol so within two minutes I had educated him and his girlfriend on everything from the endocannabinoid system that runs through all human beings and animals to how CBD regulates our homeostasis ensuring our body's self defense system against disease, illness and injury is strong.

My patient's girlfriend first compliments me on my intelligence and then her mood shifts when she says,

"You remind me of the people who kidnapped my son. They were smart like you, wore button up shirts like you are wearing... Are you one of them? Are you a part of the cult that took my son?!?"

Containing the sudden fear that washes over me I inquire,

"Your son was kidnapped? What group are you talking about? I can assure you I am not a part of any group.   I have delivered here before to your boyfriend."

She suspiciously eyes me over and says,

"He is missing and has been for a month. So are you sure you are not one of them?"

Thankfully my patient chimes in and backs me up,

"He has been here before, he is not with them. Look, he has other patients he has to deliver too..."

Before my patient can finish his girlfriend shouts,

"They could be sending people to our house to get information. Don't you understand?!? He could be one of them! My son is missing and you don't care... do you both want me to cry?!"

She turns on the waterworks like it was turning on the sink in the bathroom. My patient and I are struck by silence and we sit there with time frozen around us.

She all at once stops crying and says,

"I'm investigating here. Let me investigate."

My patient remains quiet and her focus is redirected at me. How badly I wanted to leave. I calmly respond,

"I can assure you that I have nothing to do with your son being missing and I am not a part of any group other than the company that delivers medication to your boyfriend."

She suddenly changes tune, "I know you are not one of them. You just are well educated like them and your shirt is similar to theirs."

I had been inside my patient's house for about thirty minutes. It was time to go even if it inspired tears, but she had one last request of me,

"Promise me you will look into this."

I had retrieved my case and had my back to the door before I respond to her request,

"I work ten hours a day, so I barely have time for myself, but if I get time..."

I calmly say, as my hand reaches behind me searching for the door to the outside.

The following question from her sends me into third person and I am suddenly watching the whole scene from the ceiling, as she asks again,

"Are you sure you are not one of them?"

I smile wide and meet her directly in the eyes responding with,

"Have a great day. It was really good seeing both of you and I will think positive thoughts for your son."

Still observing myself from the third person angle on the ceiling, I walk backwards through the now beautifully opened door carefully making my way down the sidewalk towards my car.

Briefly I glance over my shoulder to see her standing outside the open door with her hands on her hips and a doubtful look upon her face.

"GHOST STORY"

One particular evening, at around 10 p.m., I receive a new patient ticket. After setting my GPS, I put my car into drive and make the call to my patient. The number informs me that this phone does not have voicemail set-up so I hang up and continue towards my patient anyways.

I'm about ten minutes away and once I am five minutes from his house I try to call him one last time. Ring, ring, ring. Nothing.

The street where this new patient lives is completely blacked out. I can barely see my brand new white car after I step out of it and close the door. No porch light on and I wonder briefly if I am on the right street or at the right house.

My defenses are suddenly on guard after I retrieve my case from my trunk and I slam it shut. I walk up to the pitch black house and knock on the door loudly.

Silence. Silence up and down the street. Silence from inside the house.

I knock again loudly and after another moment of silence I start to turn to walk back to my car. It must be the wrong house. Just then the door creaks open, but just a crack. Two eyes stare back at me from the blackness and I inquire if he was my patient. My patient nods and gestures for me to come into the pitch black house.

And still no lights are turned on.

I realize after entering the house that my patient was African-American and I begin to introduce myself but he interrupts me,

"Can you please be quiet and follow me."

Not needing to hide the look of annoyance on my face, because it was far too dark for anyone to see, I follow my patient into another pitch black room which I assume is the living room and I almost retreat back the way I came when I see two white night gowns floating in mid-air near the middle of the room.

Was it apparitions or ghosts?!

I realize it was two women standing there, in bright white night gowns, silently staring at me, so I say politely,

"Good evening."

The apparitions say nothing.

My patient escorts me down a dark hallway to a dully lit room where he closes the door behind him and gestures for me to set my case on his bed. One other woman is in the room and she shows me her recommendation so I allow her to stay in the room for my visit. I began with my new patient like I always do,

"So, every driver will be different. Some driver's cases will be well stocked, depending on the day and time of day. Also, we have coupons which are…"

SCREEECH, BANG, BANG, SCRAPE

The noise is deafening and echoes through the small room making the three of us jump. All is then dead quiet.

"What was that?"

I ask, ready at any moment to defend myself, perhaps with my case.

My patient starts moving towards the door with wide-eyes and says,

"I don't know, let me go check."

My patient quickly leaves the room and shuts the door behind him.   An eternity ticks by but really only thirty seconds pass then my patient returns and informs me that everything is good, so I continue where I left off,

"So now for daily Coupons. There is the everyday coupon where you get three eighters then you get the fourth eighter for free, you can mix and match but the cheapest is always for free. Then there is the Weed Maps coupon and that changes every day so always...."

BANG BANG SCRAPE SCREEEECH BANG

The cartoon version of me would have my heart pounding out of my chest right about now with Wiley Coyote legs spinning as I create an outline of myself on the wall as I bust through it to freedom.

Instead, I calmly ask,

"Is everything ok?"

Again my patient exits and returns a minute later informing me that everything is good. I attempt to continue but before I can open my mouth...

BANG SCREECH SCREECH SCRAPE

Silence. Rinse, repeat. So I calmly inform my patient that I shall be exiting, stage left.

"I am sorry but I have to go. I am not sure what is going on but it is time to go."

Like the flash, my case is packed and my hand is turning the handle on the door to exit. The moment I open the door I come face to face with a grandmother who has scowl that would curl your hair. She is wearing a white night gown, just like the ones from the living room. I smile politely quickly saying my goodbyes as I walk down the hall towards the living room.

The whole house is still pitch black so it takes me a moment for my eyes to focus and to seek out the exit. I encounter only one night gown apparition in the living room this time but it is in different location.

I toss another "good night" over my shoulder and swiftly stride towards what appears to be where I entered. I turn the door handle and the cold air outside invades my lungs, but a hand lands on my shoulder.

I stop, plant my feet firmly in place and turn slowly around. My patient's eyes meet mine in the darkness of his living room and he says,

"Are you sure you can't stay?"

Insane laughter echoes inside my mind, so I finish with,

"Have a great night!"

I walk confidently to my car and open my trunk with my clicker and place my case inside my trunk. After calmly getting into my car I drive a couple blocks before pulling over to inform dispatch why I walked out on my patient. I then proceeded to shake like a leaf on a traumatized tree during a winter storm for the following few minutes.

The company I work for backed me up, surprisingly, and to this day that is one of the only patients I know of that was blacklisted.

"STARBUCKS LOVE OR EVOL"

Always is there a desire, a want, a need...
for caffeine. Sometimes more than food.
After ordering my piping hot caramel frap
and walking back towards my car in this
glorious ninety eight degree, in the middle
of December, Californian weather and I
began to question my choice in drinks.

"BLING BLING" which means a patient and
forward I drive with my piping hot carmel
frap.

Upon arrival, I am greeted by a very friendly
man whose neatly trimmed fiery red beard
hair almost sparkles in the sun. After
setting my case on the couch and shaking
hands with his girlfriend who exits meekly, I
begin my routine.

I go over our coupons, quickly finding what the patient is looking for has definitely become second nature now, and once I finish it is obvious my patient is content. I always aim to please.

I punch up his ticket as each of us are chatting and joking about life. Cordiality is at an all time high. Upon the final few clicks on my phone, adding in the coupons, I say,

"Alright, here is what we got with the coupons and everything added up."

I was crouching next to my patient, at an awkward angle, so I shift briefly to sit down to give him a better look at my phone. The unthinkable occurs.

TOOOOT

Yup. I tooted, farted, expelled internal gases in the most natural, but terribly embarrassing and wonderfully relieving way possible.

I imagine that any foundation for a future professional relationship is now gone with my wind, so I say what feels natural.

"Oh my."

I believe was my response. Looking back, I suppose it was naturally perfect.

I look at my patient, who looks at me with concerning eyes, and we both bust into laughter.   I apologize whole-heartedly, red-faced and quickly humbled, and my patient was beyond kind responding with,

"It is only natural."

I tacked on a few freebies to that delivery.

Despite everything I received a cash tip from the patient which was overly generous to say the least. I definitely consider it a pity tip, and I'll take it.

Thank God his girlfriend had left the room minutes before the toot.

"CLOCK OUT TIME"

For whatever reason, the most interestingly unique moments usually occur in the evenings. The closer you get to the end of your shift, the more likely something weird, scary or incredibly annoying will occur.

One such evening, as my shift was about fifteen minutes from over and eleven o'clock was about to hit, I receive one last patient. There is always a part of you, no matter how badly you might want or need tips, that thinks in these moments,

"What the !@#$. Seriously, it is almost 11 p.m.!"

I punch in the address and then call the patient to inform her I am ten minutes away. A woman with an exoticly appealing accent answers and she finishes the call with,

"I look forward to meeting you."

The street is in a nice and quiet neighborhood on the outskirts of town. The front porch light turns on after I step out of my car and walk to my trunk to retrieve my case. I note how courteous that is of her because you would be surprised how many times I arrive at pitch black houses, tripping and falling all over myself just trying to find front doors.

My patient's lawn is well landscaped and the fragrance of roses fills the walkway to her door. Just as I near the front door it opens, revealing a very well tanned woman with long, wet flowing black hair and who is wearing a pink bathrobe. She appears to have just gotten out of the shower.

Somehow maintaining my professionalism and where my eyes should focus upon, I shake her hand and introduce myself. She invites me inside and asks if I would like anything to drink, perhaps tea. I politely decline.

My patient and I cordially banter as I open my case and I set it on the living room table. I kneel on the ground, providing her the position of power, and she sits on the table in front of me and next to my case. She crosses her legs and rubs her hands together,

"Mmmm, everything looks so good."

I did not disagree.

Her eyes scan over my case and she asks me what I'd recommend for body pains but without having the "couch lock" effects. Her accent sounds so beautiful when she speaks especially coming from her plump lips. I had to remind myself to focus on the job at hand.

"This Redwood O.G. is a beautiful strain. It has tasty earthiness all the way through the smoke, it has very relaxing effects and not any couch lock, and it has rock hard buds so the bowls last a long time. Here smell for yourself."

I pop the top of the bottle and hold it under her nose. Even though the Redwood O.G. immediately fills the room with its earthy aroma, all I can smell is the fragrance of my patient's shampoo, or lotion, or perfurme.

"Ohhh. You are right, that is good. Rock hard too! My favorite,"

My patient said, as she plucks a nug from the bottle and squeezes the sticky nug in-between her fingers. She puts the nug back into the bottle and then puts her fingers in her mouth, one by one, to suck off the sticky THC crystals that got stuck upon them.

"You have good tastes," she said, as she finishes licking her fingers.

The blackness of her pupils for a moment seems to swallow me whole. I take a slow deep breathe, responding sternly and with a smile,

"I try."

The fragrance of her shampoo, or lotion, or whatever that unbelievable alluring scent was gloriously is overwhelming, but I remind myself that I must maintain professionalism.

"So am I your last patient of the night?"

I confirm her question with a nod, as I focus on the task of punching up her ticket on my phone. She uncrosses and re-crosses her legs and the asks me,

"What are you doing after this? Any plans?"

I briefly pause, my brain apparently rebooting, yet my eyes and ears still functioning quite flawlessly,

"No, no plans. Haven't had any plans in years it seems. Not since my divorce when I gave my X everything and took nothing. Just ten hours a day, working, bringing people relief."

I think to myself how moronic I just sounded and wonder why I even said all that. God I'm such a putz.

I show her the breakdown of her ticket on my phone and the couple coupons I applied to save her quite a decent amount of money. I tossed in a free edible because... well, she deserved it.

My patient rises from the table, bathrobe shimmering, turns around and walks towards her purse that is resting on the ground next to her entertainment center. Bending over, she not hastily retrieves the donation from her purse.

I stare quickly down at my phone yet my peripherals prevail. Deep, deep inside, I sigh.

She rises with the donation in hand and I begin packing up my case. Just as I slide my case into its sheath, my attention is suddenly focused upon that ever-present sweet fragrance that again invades my senses.

I glance up to find directly in front of me that shimmering pink bathrobe, slightly parted in all the most mysteriously shadowy places, with well rounded, smooth and shiny legs peaking out at me, so tan and shiny I actually see my own reflection in them.

I clear my throat, rising to meet her abyss-like gaze. She hands me the donation and asks,

"Do you accept tips?"

I smile and nod,

"Of course. We are hourly paid so tips mean the world to us drivers."

She hands me a twenty dollar bill and I thank her extensively, finishing with,

"Your beauty alone would have been the highlight to my day, but this works too."

Her laugh is as wonderful as her accent, and just as appealing as her fragrance.

"You're funny... and smart... and kind,"

She says, as she follows close behind me and as I near her front door I turn and say,

"Thank you. I do my best. It was a pleasure meeting you and I hope the rest of your night goes well. I am sure it will now."

She frowns, which is somehow sadly beautiful, and says,

"I am just going to be here all by myself, with my meds. Just missing one thing."

I look at her and ask,

"What's that?"

She smiles.

This is when I clocked out for the evening.

"PACK MENTALITY"

A fellow driver who has delivered for over four years told me this story about a very tense situation he was involved in and I will recount the story in first person.

It was mid-afternoon when I arrived at my patient's second floor apartment in Vista, California. There were obviously numerous people inside the apartment because I could hear them hooting and hollering as I walked up the stairs.

Immediately upon knocking, the door shot open and I was energetically invited inside by an individual who was not my patient. The apartment was a tiny two bedroom, one bathroom apartment that was maybe about seven hundred square feet and within this tiny living quarters was crammed six very athletic men who were watching football.

I asked my patient where to put my case to which he gestured to the small crate in the middle of the tiny room. After setting my case down and checking his paperwork I inform my patient,

"Before I can start is there either a room we can go into or where your friend's can chill for a minute while we go over the case? Legalities, I'm sure you understand."

Unfortunately there was very little understanding with this particular crowd and someone responded with,

"Ahhhh man. Come on, why can't we all stay?! Come on man, we won't tell anyone. That isn't cool bro."

I politely smile and show a little leniency, so I tell them that they can only stay if they have their marijuana recommendations with them. The group of guys all vocally express their disappointment as my patient and I rise to leave the room. A few of these comments were "You aren't cool" and a few even went so far to "boo" me. That was a first.

After finishing with my patient, who was beyond happy with all the coupons and savings he made, I packed up my case and made my way out of the room and as I passed by the crowd of men in the living room they once again assaulted me with a chorus of "boo's" as I left. I was greatly relieved to be out of that place.

Thankfully, this was the only time in years I was boo'ed by people at a delivery.

"GRANDMA JANE"

A fellow driver received a call from a patient an hour after delivering to her. This adorable ninety-year old patient called to update the driver on her opinion of his opinion about the products acquired through his recommendation.

This patient is barely able to move around her big house by herself and has some ailment that makes her suffer greatly. She is a favorite among the drivers and she never tips, which she makes up for with her warm personality. We will nickname this patient "Grandma Jane" for the sake of this story.

This particular driver received Grandma Jane's call while with another patient so naturally he let the call go to voicemail.

Rarely will we receive a call from a patient after the delivery has occurred and if we do, it is only when something has gone wrong. Usually some issue requiring resolution and rarely is it convenient.

This call, however, was not the case.

The driver saved the message and played it for me about a week later and it went like this:

In the softest and kindest grandma voice imaginable,

"Hellooooo! I just ate my brownie that you recommended after finishing all of my supper, so I ate it for dessert. Boy was it yummy! And well, I know you said that it was Indica and would make me tired, but I don't think it is Indica, because I'm very chatty right now and I feel absolutely wonderful!!"

At this point in the message a series of grandma giggles can be heard which sounded kind of like,

"Hehehehehe."

Grandma Jane finishes the message with,

"I just wanted to say thank you for your recommendations and God Bless you, and all that you do! Oh I just love these brownies. Good night!"

"DOWN BOY, WHOA BOY"

In almost a year of delivering medical marijuana to patients I have never had a tense or dangerous moment with any animal. I always considered it a privilege that I grew up with dogs and others animals and I feel I understand dogs on a deeper level.

Upon arriving at my patient's house, just on the border of the Camp Pendleton military base, I immediately notice the numerous signs on the fences and windows warning people of the "Killer Dog" that resided there. I thought nothing of it and opened the gate making my way to the front door.

A bell on the gate rang loudly notifying people from far and wide that I had entered the yard. Like cannons firing off during Camp Pendleton's training drills combined with the impact of the shells were comparable to the woofs of this beautiful white Pit-Bull.

I was asked to wait outside while he put the dog away but he returned with it still jumping at his back.

After inviting me inside and making my way to the living room, my patient was constantly in between his dog and I. We will call the dog Killer for the duration.

Killer very persistently lunges at me quite a few times while my patient pushes at him and yells,

"Whoa! Calm down killer."

After punching in everything my patient wanted into my I-Pad, I stood up and snagged the donation from my patient. I begin packing up my case and exchanging farewells when Killer gives me a farewell of his own.

Killer hops onto the back of my leg and starts going to town. My patient attempts to pull Killer from my leg but Killer is intent on maintaining his position of power.

Finally my patient pulls his dog off and apologizes,

"Sorry, he never does that."

Before I could reply, Killer breaks free from my patient's grip and is back up on my leg giving it another once over. After another tug-of-war with his dog I recovered my leg and made my way to the door while my patient held back Killer with difficulty.

It is with great sadness that I say that my leg was never the same again after that delivery and the pants... well I heard that the pants spontaneously combusted a few days later in a hunting accident.

"TAILGATING"

Two hours left, in what seemed like a ten hour day that would never friggin' end. I was fortunate though that my route for the day was near where I lived so once my phone quieted up I dared race home briefly for some food and relief.

Only minutes on the freeway, I reached my exit and just as I came to a stop at the red light ahead I realized the car in front of me was a police cruiser.

This happens just about every day and even though it is nothing new there is always a tension that is inspired by their presence. There appears to be a public consensus these days about police in that they make us feel more tense and uncomfortable, instead of making us feel protected and safe when they are in the vicinity. This is a sad, unfortunate societal truth, at least in my mind.

The light went from red to green and I kept a good car length distance from the police cruise as we veered left onto the crowded parkway. After passing through two green lights, in less than half a block, traffic came to another halt at a red light and I came to a complete stop behind the police cruiser.

It was a four lane road and I was in one of the right lanes behind the police cruiser when I realize that the far left lane ahead is a turning lane and would soon have a green light with only one red dominoes delivery car waiting for that left turn.

I put on my signal for the left lane, checked over my shoulder, my mirrors, and I pulled into the left turning lane and a few seconds later I came to a complete stop behind the red dominoes delivery car.

The police cruiser suddenly appears behind me and comes to a stop.

Quite a few things flash through my mind,

"I didn't do anything wrong. I have all my paperwork. I'm starving. I wouldn't mind some Dominoes pizza. Naw, I hate Dominoes."

The light turns green and the Dominoes delivery guy turns left and then comes to a complete stop needing to immediately turn right into the complex where the Dominoes pizza building is located. I stop, allowing little red rover to move on over and I then proceed steadily down the pitch black road out of the city and into the suburbs with the police cruiser in hot pursuit.

After a block I turn on my signal to turn right, come to a complete stop at a stop sign and the police cruiser comes to a complete stop with me. I proceed to make my right turn and the police cruiser lights me up.

Dramatic red and blue rave lights pierce the night and I turn onto the first street I come across. Joy Court. How appropriate.

After retrieving my insurance and drivers license I wait for the officer and the first thing he says as he walks up is,

"Whew, it smells like weed. Do you have marijuana in the car Sir?"

Stunned for some reason, I stupidly say while holding my insurance and drivers license out in the air at the officer,

"I have my California state-issued medical marijuana card."

With the light blinding me the officer responds to my stupidity,

"That is not what I asked. Please do not be evasive Sir. Do you have marijuana in your car?"

Shaking my head, I politely say,

"No. It is in my trunk. Here, I think this is everything you should need."

I reach into the backseat of my car for my tiny black folder of legal documents and in the back of my head I picture the police officer pulling his gun on me instinctively ending me.

Thankfully, I am quicker on the draw and before the officer says,

"Please keep your hands where I can see them."

I have extracted my folder and have opened it to display the documents that are now required.

"I work for a collective and I deliver medications to confirmed legally licensed patients. Everything you need should be right there."

The officer says nothing while slowly flipping through the powerful tiny black binder, as if he has become entranced. Power stripped away. Closing the binder, the officer looks up and asks me,

"Do you know why I pulled you over?"

I smile meekly and again stupidly respond,

"I wasn't speeding... and I know I came to a complete stop at that stop sign, so I'm not sure."

Again the blinding light of his flashlight in my eyes and finally the reason for the officer having this lovely discussion with me on this dark lonely road was revealed, which was,

"Tailgating. You were tailgating me off the freeway and you tailgated that red car."

My blank stare said it all, but I said,

"Uhhh, ok. I see."

The officer takes my binder, insurance and both identifications leaving me to the solitude of my car and the insanely stroke-inducing red and blue rave lights that never end. I pick up my phone and inform dispatch of the situation and for them to hand off my patients to another driver for the rest of the night because I was clocking out early tonight. I couldn't wait for this debacle to be finally over and I was either home, safe, or in jail, screwed.

Thoughts of being arrested, despite being legally licensed, floated in and out of my mind. In-N-Out floated into my mind and sounded much better than my current situation.

Finally, the officer returned after a nice quick thirty minute wait, binder in hand.

"Everything's in order. All I need to do is see the contents of your trunk. Do I have your permission to search your car and trunk?"

I open the door to my car and step out,

"Of course, be my guest. There's no weapons, or anything."

I walk around to the back of my car to pop my trunk and am greeted by six police officers with three newly arrived cop cars lighting up the peaceful night. My trunk opens revealing an extremely well organized trunk with my case and back stock stacked like a Tetris pro.

"Wow. So this is it?"

The officer asks while looking into one of my coolers briefly while the numerous police cruisers lights proceed to lull me into a epileptic seizure.

"Yup. That's my case that I take into my patient's house, so they can pick out their meds and that is the little bit of back stock I have."

The officer steps back and asks me to put my case onto his hood and display the contents to which I comply. After pulling out the case from the sheath I take this opportunity to educate the uneducated.

Besides, I was doing nothing else better at that particular moment and I had nowhere else to go.

"These products are CBD-only products and contain no THC, so there is no medicating affect, or high to them. CBD regulates our homeostasis in all our endocannabinoid systems and the last time we consumed CBD was in breast milk as a child. This here is a one month supply CBD sublingual eye dropper and one of these should be in every household, in my opinion."

The cops sat there slack jawed as I force fed them the information and each time my hand waivered over a product in my case at least two of the officers would place their hand on the gun attached to the belts around their waist.

"Aren't you afraid of carrying all this and getting robbed?"

While I think to myself,

"No, I only worry about the people who question if I worry."

In reality, I respond with a different truthful answer,

"No. I trust my patients."

The officer pulls out a camera and snaps pictures of my trunk, my case and lucky me, me. Displaying his ticket book, the officer asks me to sign the ticket which only has the citation of tailgating.

"I could have put on the ticket that you didn't come to a complete stop at that stop sign, but I'm cutting you a break."

I smile politely at the officers, thank them for their time and wish them a good evening.

A few months later I schedule my trial to contest my two hundred and fifty four dollar tailgating ticket.

I arrive at the court in my suit and tie at 8 a.m. and I have everything I'm going to ask the officer lined up in my mind.

The judge calls my case second out of a packed courtroom and when the officer is called to present himself, silence fills the courtroom.

Is this what justice sounds like? An absentee kind of quiet.

My two hundred and fifty four dollar tailgating ticket was dismissed and I proceeded to have a very good day.

www.ingramcontent.com/pod-product-compliance
Lightning Source LLC
Chambersburg PA
CBHW072134280526
45788CB00002B/635